Home Remedies: How to Become Your Own Home Doctor

A Complete Guide to Home Remedies

By: Stacey L. Reid

9781631871627

I0413989

PUBLISHERS NOTES

Disclaimer – Speedy Publishing, LLC

This publication is intended to provide helpful and informative material. It is not intended to diagnose, treat, cure, or prevent any health problem or condition, nor is intended to replace the advice of a physician. No action should be taken solely on the contents of this book. Always consult your physician or qualified health-care professional on any matters regarding your health and before adopting any suggestions in this book or drawing inferences from it.

The author and publisher specifically disclaim all responsibility for any liability, loss or risk, personal or otherwise, which is incurred as a consequence, directly or indirectly, from the use or application of any contents of this book.

Any and all product names referenced within this book are the trademarks of their respective owners. None of these owners have sponsored, authorized, endorsed, or approved this book.

Always read all information provided by the manufacturers' product labels before using their products. The author and publisher are not responsible for claims made by manufacturers.

This book was originally printed before 2014. This is an adapted reprint by Speedy Publishing, LLC with newly updated content designed to help readers with much more accurate and timely information and data.

Speedy Publishing, LLC

40 E Main Street,

Newark

Delaware

19711

Contact Us: 1-888-248-4521

Website: http://www.speedypublishing.com

REPRINTED Paperback Edition: ISBN: 9781631871627

Manufactured in the United States of America

DEDICATION

This book is dedicated to my husband who is my greatest source of support. He gives advice when he needs to and no matter what he encourages me to keep on working for what I want.

TABLE OF CONTENTS

CHAPTER 1- WHAT CAUSES DISEASE

"Toxemia is the basic cause of all so-called diseases.

In the process of tissue-building (metabolism), there is cell-building (anabolism) and cell destruction (catabolism). The broken-down tissue is toxic. In the healthy body (when nerve energy is normal), this toxic material is eliminated from the blood as fast as it is evolved. But when nerve energy is dissipated from any cause (such as physical or mental excitement or bad habits) the body becomes weakened or enervated. When the body is enervated, elimination is checked. This, in turn, results in retention of toxins in the blood-- the condition which we speak of as toxemia.

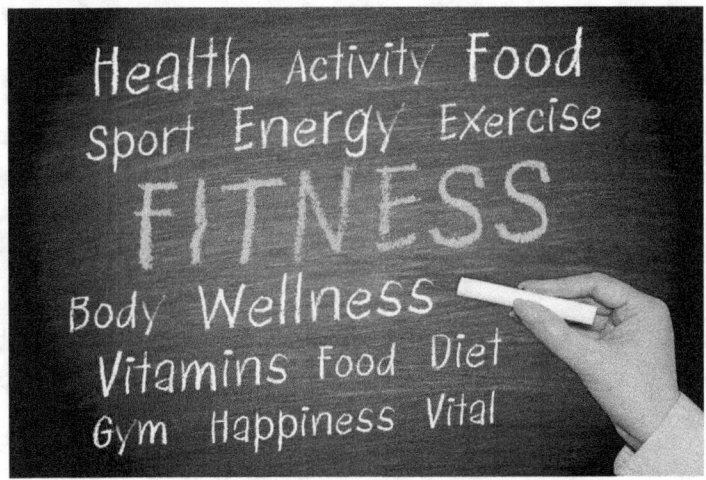

This state produces a crisis which is nothing more than heroic or extraordinary efforts by the body to eliminate waste or toxin from the blood. It is this crisis which we term disease. Such accumulation of toxin when once established will continue until nerve energy has been restored to normal by removing the cause.

Home Remedies

So-called disease is nature's effort to eliminate toxin from the blood. All so-called diseases are crises of toxemia." _John H. Tilden, M.D., Toxemia Explained._ Toxins are divided into two groups; namely exogenous, those formed in the alimentary canal from fermentation and decomposition following imperfect or faulty digestion. If the fermentation is of vegetables or fruit, the toxins are irritating, stimulating and enervating, but not so dangerous or destructive to organic life as putrefaction, which is a fermentation set up in nitrogenous matter--protein-bearing foods, but particularly animal foods. Endogenous toxins are auto generated. They are the waste products of metabolism. _Dr. John. H. Tilden, Impaired Health: Its Cause and Cure, 1921._

Suppose a fast-growing city is having traffic jams. "We don't like it!" protest the voters. "Why are these problems happening?" asks the city council, trying to look like they are doing something about it.

Experts then proffer answers. "Because there are too many cars," says the Get A Horse Society. The auto makers suggest it is because there are uncoordinated traffic lights and because almost all the businesses send their employees home at the same time. Easy to fix!

And no reason whatsoever to limit the number of cars. The asphalt industry suggests it is because the size and amount of roads is inadequate.

What do we do then? Tax cars severely until few can afford them? Legislate opening and closing hours of businesses to stagger to'ing and fro'ing? Hire a smarter municipal highway engineer to synchronize the traffic lights? Build larger and more efficient streets? Demand that auto companies make cars smaller so more can fit the existing roads? Tax gasoline prohibitively, pass out and give away free bicycles in virtually unlimited quantities while simultaneously building mass rail systems? What? Which?

When we settle on a solution we have simultaneously chosen what we consider the real, underlying cause of the problem. If our chosen reason was the real reason then our solution results in a real cure. If we picked wrongly, our attempt at solution may result in no cure, or create a worse situation than we had before.

The American Medical Association style of medicine (a philosophy I will henceforth call allopathic) has a model that explains the causes of illness. It suggests that anyone who is sick is a victim. Either they were attacked by a "bad" organism--virus, bacteria, yeast, pollen, cancer cell, etc.--or they have a "bad" organ--liver, kidney, gall bladder, even brain. Or, the victim may also have been cursed by bad genes. In any case, the cause of the disease is not the person and the person is neither responsible for creating their own complaint nor is the victim capable of making it go away. This institutionalized irresponsibility seems useful for both parties to the illness, doctor and patient. The patient is not required to do anything about their complaint except pay (a lot) and obediently follow the instructions of the doctor, submitting unquestioningly to their drugs and surgeries. The physician then acquires a role of being considered vital to the survival of others and thus obtains great status, prestige, authority, and financial remuneration.

Perhaps because the sick person is seen to have been victimized, and it is logically impossible to consider a victimizer as anything but something evil, the physician's cure is often violent, confrontational. Powerful poisons are used to rejigger body chemistry or to arrest the multiplication of disease bacteria or to suppress symptoms; if it is possible to sustain life without them, "bad," poorly-functioning organs are cut out.

I've had a lot of trouble with the medical profession. Over the years doctors have made attempts to put me in jail and keep me in fear. But they never stopped me. When I've had a client die there has been an almost inevitable coroner's investigation, complete with detectives and the sheriff. Fortunately, I practice in rural Oregon, where the local people have a deeply-held belief in individual liberty and where the authorities know they would have had a very hard time finding a jury to convict me. Had I chosen to practice with a high profile and had I located Great Oaks School of Health in a major market area where the physicians were able to charge top dollar, I probably would have spent years behind bars as did other heroes of my profession such as Linda Hazzard and Royal Lee.

So I have acquired an uncomplimentary attitude about medical doctors, a viewpoint I am going to share with you urgently, despite the fact that doing so will alienate some of my readers. But I do so because most Americans are entirely enthralled by doctors, and this doctor-god worship kills a lot of them.

However, before I get started on the medicos, let me state that one area exists where I do have fundamental admiration for allopathic medicine. This is its handling of trauma. I agree that a body can become the genuine victim of fast moving bullets. It can be innocently cut, smashed, burned, crushed and broken. Trauma are not diseases and modern medicine has become quite skilled at putting traumatized bodies back together. Genetic abnormality may be another undesirable physical condition that is beyond the purview of natural medicine. However, the expression of contra-survival genetics can often be controlled by nutrition. And the expression of poor genetics often results from poor nutrition, and thus is similar to a degenerative disease condition, and thus is well within the scope of natural medicine.

Today's suffering American public is firmly in the AMA's grip. People have been effectively prevented from learning much about medical alternatives, have been virtually brainwashed by clever media management that portrays other medical models as dangerous and/or ineffective. Legislation influenced by the allopathic doctors' union, the American Medical Association, severely limits or prohibits the practice of holistic health. People are repeatedly directed by those with authority to an allopathic doctor whenever they have a health problem, question or confusion.

Other types of healers are considered to be at best harmless as long as they confine themselves to minor complaints; at worst, when naturopaths, hygienists, or homeopaths seek to treat serious disease conditions they are called quacks, accused of unlicensed practice of medicine and if they persist or develop a broad, successful, high-profile and (this is the very worst) profitable practice, they are frequently jailed.

Even licensed MDs are crushed by the authorities if they offer non-standard treatments. So when anyone seeks an alternative health approach it is usually because their complaint has already failed to vanish after consulting a whole series of allopathic doctors. This highly unfortunate kind of sufferer not only has a degenerative condition to rectify, they may have been further damaged by harsh medical treatments and additionally, they have a considerable amount of brainwashing to overcome.

The AMA has succeeded at making their influence over information and media so pervasive that most people do not even realize that the doctors' union is the source of their medical outlook. Whenever an American complains of some malady, a concerned and honestly caring friend will demand to know have they yet consulted a medical doctor.

Failure to do so on one's own behalf is considered highly irresponsible. Concerned relatives of seriously ill adults who decline standard medical therapy may, with a great show of self-righteousness, have the sick person judged mentally incompetent so that treatment can be forced upon them. When a parent fails to seek standard medical treatment for their child, the adult may well be found guilty of criminal negligence, raising the interesting issue of who "owns" the child, the parents or the State.

It is perfectly acceptable to die while under conventional medical care. Happens all the time, in fact but holistic alternatives are represented as stupidly risky, especially for serious conditions such as cancer. People with cancer see no choice but to do chemotherapy, radiation, and radical surgery because this is the current allopathic medical approach. On some level people may know that these remedies are highly dangerous but they have been told by their attending oncologist that violent therapies are their only hope of survival, however poor that may be. If a cancer victim doesn't proceed immediately with such treatment their official prognosis becomes worse by the hour.

Such scare tactics are common amongst the medical profession, and they leave the recipient so terrified that they meekly and obediently give up all self-determinism, sign the liability waiver, and submit, no questions asked. Many then die after suffering intensely from the therapy, long before the so-called disease could have actually caused their demise. I will later offer alternative and frequently successful (but not guaranteed) approaches to treating cancer that do not require the earliest-possible detection, surgery or poisons.

If holistic practitioners were to apply painful treatments like allopaths use, ones with such poor statistical outcomes like allopaths use, there would most certainly be witch hunts and all such irresponsible, greedy quacks would be safely imprisoned. I find it highly ironic that for at least the past twenty five hundred years the basic principle of good medicine has been that the treatment must first do no harm. This is such an obvious truism that even the AMA doctors pledge to do the same thing when they take the Hippocratic Oath. Yet virtually every action taken by the allopath is a conscious compromise between the potential harm of the therapy and its potential benefit.

In absolute contrast, if a person dies while on a natural hygiene program, they died because their end was inevitable no matter what therapy was attempted. Almost certainly receiving hygienic therapy contributed to making their last days far more comfortable and relatively free of pain without using opiates. I have personally taken on clients sent home to die after they had suffered everything the doctors could do to them, told they had only a few days, weeks, or months to live. Some of these clients survived as a result of hygienic programs even at that late date. And some didn't. The amazing thing was that any of them survived at all, because the best time to begin a hygienic program is as early in the degenerative process as possible, not after the body has been drastically weakened by invasive and toxic treatments. Later on, I'll tell you about some of these cases.

Something I consider especially ironic is that when the patient of a medical doctor dies, it is inevitably thought that the blessed doctor did all that could be done; rarely is any blame laid. If the physician was especially careless or stupid, their fault can only result in a civil suit, covered by malpractice insurance. But let a holistic practitioner treat a sick person and have that person follow any of their suggestions or take any natural remedies and have that person die or worsen and it instantly becomes the natural doctor's fault. Great blame is placed and the practitioner faces inquests, grand juries, manslaughter charges, jail time and civil suits that can't be insured against.

Home Remedies

Allopathic medicine rarely makes a connection between the real causes of a degenerative or infectious disease and its cure. The causes are usually considered mysterious: we don't know why the pancreas is acting up, etc. The sick are sympathized with as victims who did nothing to contribute to their condition. The cure is a highly technical battle against the illness, whose weapons are defined in Latin and far beyond the understanding of a layperson.

Hygienic medicine presents an opposite view. To the naturopath, illness is not a perplexing and mysterious occurrence over which you have no control or understanding. The causes of disease are clear and simple, the sick person is rarely a victim of circumstance and the cure is obvious and within the competence of a moderately intelligent sick person themselves to understand and help administer. In natural medicine, disease is a part of living that you are responsible for, and quite capable of handling.

Asserting that the sick are pitiable victims is financially beneficial to doctors. It makes medical intervention seem a vital necessity for every ache and pain. It makes the sick become dependent. I'm not implying that most doctors knowingly are conniving extortionists. Actually most medical doctors are genuinely well-intentioned. I've also noticed that most medical doctors are at heart very timid individuals who consider that possession of a MD degree and license proves that they are very important, proves them to be highly intelligent, even makes them fully qualified to pontificate on many subjects not related to medicine at all.

Doctors obtain an enormous sense of self-importance at medical school, where they proudly endured the high pressure weeding out of any free spirit unwilling to grind away into the night for seven or more years. Anyone incapable of absorbing and regurgitating huge amounts of rote information; anyone with a disrespectful or irreverent attitude toward the senior doctor-gods who arrogantly serve as med school professors, anyone like this was eliminated with especial rapidity. When the thoroughly submissive, homogenized survivors are finally licensed, they assume the status of junior doctor-gods.

But becoming an official medical deity doesn't permit one to create their own methods. The AMA's professional oversight and control system makes continued possession of the license to practice (and the high income that usually comes with it) entirely dependent on continued conformity to what is defined by the AMA as "correct practice." Any doctor who innovates beyond strict limits or uses non-standard treatments is in real danger of losing their livelihood and status.

Not only are licensed graduates of AMA-sanctioned medical schools kept on a very tight leash, doctors of other persuasions who use other methods to heal the sick or help them heal themselves are persecuted and prosecuted. Extension of the AMA's control through regulatory law and police power is justified in the name of preventing quackery and making sure the ignorant and gullible public receives only scientifically proven effective medical care.

Those on the other side of the fence view the AMA's oppression as an effective way to make sure the public has no real choices but to use union doctors, pay their high fees and suffer greatly by misunderstanding of the true cause of disease and its proper cure.

If there are any actual villains responsible for this suppressive tragedy some of them are to be found in the inner core of the AMA, officials who may perhaps fully and consciously comprehend the suppressive system they promulgate.

Hygienists usually inform the patient quite clearly and directly that the practitioner has no ability to heal them or cure their condition and that no doctor of any type actually is able to heal. Only the body can heal itself, something it is eager and usually very able to do if only given the chance. One pithy old saying among hygienists goes, "if the body can't heal itself, nothing can heal it." The primary job of the hygienic practitioner is to reeducate the patient by conducting them through their first natural healing process. If this is done well the sick person learns how to get out of their own body's way and permit its native healing power to manifest. Unless later the victim of severe traumatic injury, never again will that person need obscenely expensive medical procedures. Hygienists rarely make six figure incomes from regular, repeat business.

This aspect of hygienic medicine makes it different than almost all the others, even most other holistic methods. Hygiene is the only system that does not interpose the assumed healing power of a doctor between the patient and wellness. When I was younger and less experienced I thought that the main reason traditional medical practice did not stress the body's own healing power and represented the doctor as a necessary intervention was for profit. But after practicing for over twenty years I now understand that the last thing most people want to hear is that their own habits, especially their eating patterns and food choices, are responsible for their disease and that their cure is to only be accomplished through dietary reform, which means unremittingly applied self-discipline.

One of the hardest things to ask of a person is to change a habit.

The reason that AMA doctors have most of the patients is they're giving the patients exactly what they want, which is to be allowed to continue in their unconscious irresponsibility.

The Cause of Disease

Ever since natural medicine arose in opposition to the violence of so-called scientific medicine, every book on the subject of hygiene, once it gets past its obligatory introductions and warm ups, must address The Cause of Disease. This is a required step because we see the cause of disease and its consequent cure in a very different manner than the allopath. Instead of many causes, we see one basic reason why. Instead of many unrelated cures, we have basically one approach to fix all ills that can be fixed.

A beautiful fifty cent word that means a system for explaining something is paradigm, pronounced paradigm. I am fond of this word because it admits the possibility of many differing yet equally true explanations for the same reality. Of all available paradigms, Natural Hygiene suits me best and has been the one I've used for most of my career.

The Natural Hygienist's paradigm for the cause of both degenerative and infectious disease is called the Theory of Toxemia, or "self-poisoning."

Before explaining this theory it will help many readers if I digress a brief moment about the nature and validity of alternative paradigms. Not too many decades ago, scientists thought that reality was a singular, real, perpetual--that Natural Law existed much as a tree or a rock existed. In physics, for example, the mechanics of Newton were considered capital "T" True, the only possible paradigm. Any other view, not being True, was False. There was capital "N" natural capital "L" law.

More recently, great uncertainty has entered science; it has become indisputable that a theory or explanation of reality is only true only to the degree it seems to work; conflicting or various explanations can all work, all can be "true." At least, this uncertainty has overtaken the hard, physical sciences. It has not yet done so with medicine. The AMA is convinced (or is working hard to convince everyone else) that its paradigm, the allopathic approach, is Truth, is scientific, and therefore, anything else is Falsehood, is irresponsibility, is a crime against the sick.

But the actual worth or truth of any paradigm is found not in its "reality," but in its utility. Does an explanation or theory allow a person to manipulate experience and create a desired outcome. To the extent a paradigm does that, it can be considered valuable. Judged by this standard, the Theory of Toxemia must be far truer than the hodgepodge of pseudoscience taught in medical schools. Keep that in mind the next time some officious medical doctor disdainfully informs you that Theory of Toxemia was disproven in 1927 by Doctors Jeckel and Hyde.

Chapter 2- All About Fasting

The accelerated healing process that occurs during fasting can scarcely be believed by a person who has not fasted. No matter how gifted the writer, the experiential reality of fasting cannot be communicated. The great novelist Upton Sinclair wrote a book about fasting and it failed to convince the multitudes. But once a person has fasted long enough to be certain of what their own body can do to fix itself, they acquire a degree of independence little known today. Many of those experienced with fasting no longer dread being without health insurance and feel far less need for a doctor or of having a regular checkup. They know with certainty that if something degenerates in their body, their own body can fix it by itself.

Like Upton Sinclair and many others who largely failed before me, I am going to try to convince you of the virtues of fasting by urging you to try fasting yourself. If you will but try you will be changed for the better for the rest of your life. If you do not try, you will never Know.

To prompt your first step on this health-freedom road, I ask you to please carefully consider the importance of this fact: the body's routine energy budget includes a very large allocation for the daily digestion and assimilation of the food you eat. You may find my estimate surprising, but about one-third of a fairly sedentary person's entire energy consumption goes into food processing. Other uses for the body's energy include the creation or rebuilding of tissues, detoxification, moving (walking, running, etc.), talking, producing hormones, etc. Digestion is one aspect of the body's efforts that we can readily control, it is the key to having or losing health.

Home Remedies
The Effort of Digestion

Digestion is a huge, unappreciated task, unappreciated because few of us are aware of its happening in the same way we are aware of making efforts to use our voluntary muscles when working or exercising. Digestion begins in the mouth with thorough chewing. If you don't think chewing is effort, try making coleslaw in your own mouth. Chew up at least half a big head of cabbage and three big carrots that have not been shredded. Grind each bit until it liquefies and has been thoroughly mixed with saliva. I guarantee that if you even finish the chore your jaw will be tired and you will have lost all desire to eat anything else, especially if it requires chewing.

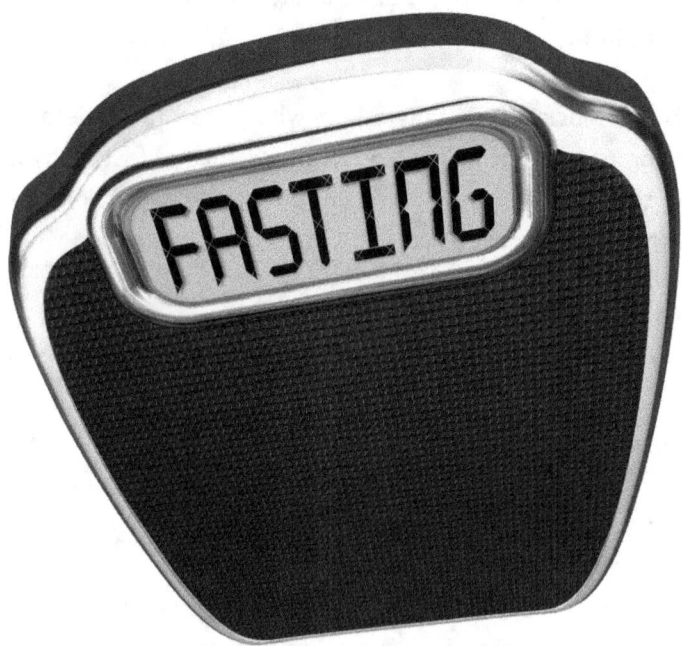

Making the saliva you just used while chewing the cabbage is by itself, a huge and unappreciated chemical effort.

Once in the stomach, chewed food has to be churned in order to mix it with hydrochloric acid, pepsin, and other digestive enzymes.

Manufacturing these enzymes is also considerable work! Churning is even harder work than chewing but normally, people are unaware of its happening. While the stomach is churning (like a washing machine) a large portion of the blood supply is redirected from the muscles in the extremities to the stomach and intestines to aid in this process. Anyone who has tried to go for a run, or take part in any other strenuous physical activity immediately after a large meal feels like a slug and wonders why they just can't make their legs move the way they usually do. So, to assist the body while it is digesting, it is wise to take a siesta as los Latinos do instead of expecting the blood to be two places at once like los norteamericanos.

After the stomach is through churning, the partially digested food is moved into the small intestine where it is mixed with more pancreatin secreted by the pancreas, and with bile from the gall bladder. Pancreatin further solubilizes proteins. Bile aids in the digestion of fatty foods. Manufacturing bile and pancreatic enzymes is also a lot of effort. Only after the carbohydrates (starches and sugars), proteins and fats have been broken down into simpler water soluble food units such as simple sugars, amino acids and fatty acids, can the body pass these nutrients into the blood thorough the little projections in the small intestines called villi.

The leftovers, elements of the food that can't be solubilized plus some remaining liquids, are passed into the large intestine. There, water and the vital mineral salts dissolved in that water, are extracted and absorbed into the blood stream through thin permeable membranes. Mucous is also secreted in the large intestine to facilitate passage of the dryish remains. This is an effort. (Intestinal mucous can become a route of secondary elimination, especially during fasting. While fasting, it is essential to take steps to expel toxic mucous in the colon before the poisons are reabsorbed.) The final residue, now called fecal matter, is squeezed along the length of the large intestines and passes out the rectum.

If all the digestive processes have been efficient there now are an abundance of soluble nutrients for the blood stream to distribute to hungry cells throughout the body. It is important to understand the process at least on the level of oversimplification just presented in order to begin to understand better how health is lost or regained through eating, digestion, and elimination. And most importantly, through not eating.

How Fasting Heals

It's an old hygienic maxim that the doctor does not heal, the medicines do not heal, only the body heals itself. If the body can't heal then nothing can heal it. The body always knows best what it needs and what to do.

But healing means repairing damaged organs and tissues and this takes energy, while a sick body is already enervated, weakened and not coping with its current stressors. If the sick person could but somehow increase the body's energy resources sufficiently, then a slowly healing body could heal faster while a worsening one, or one that was failing or one that was not getting better might heal.

Fasting does just that. To whatever degree food intake is reduced the body's digestive workload is proportionately reduced and it will naturally and far more intelligently than any physician could order, redirect energy to wherever it decides that energy is most needed. A fasting body begins accessing nutritional reserves (vitamins and minerals) previously stored in the tissues and starts converting body fat into sugar for energy fuel. During a time of water fasting, sustaining the body's entire energy and nutritional needs from reserves and fat does require a small effort, but far less effort than eating. I would guess a fasting body used about five percent of its normal daily energy budget on nutritional concerns rather than the 33 percent it needs to process new food.

Thus, water fasting puts something like 28 percent more energy at the body's disposal. This is true even though the water faster may feel weak, energyless.

I would worry if sick or toxic fasters did not complain about their weakness. They should expect to feel energyless. In fact, the more internal healing and detoxification the body requires, the tireder the faster feels because the body is very hard at work internally. A great deal of the body's energy will go toward boosting the immune system if the problem is an infection. Liberated energy can also be used for healing damaged parts, rebuilding failing organs, for breaking down and eliminating deposits of toxic materials. Only after most of the healing has occurred does a faster begin to feel energetic again. Don't expect to feel anything but tired and weak.

The only exception to this would be a person who has already significantly detoxified and healed their body by previous fasting, or the rare soul that has gone from birth through adulthood enjoying extraordinarily good nutrition and without experiencing the stressors of improper digestion. When one experienced faster I know finds himself getting "run down" or catching a cold, he quits eating until he feels really well. Instead of feeling weak as most fasters do, as each of the first four or five days of water fasting pass, he experiences a resurgence of more and more energy.

On the first fasting day he would usually feel rotten, which was why he started fasting in the first place. On the second fasting day he'd feel more alert and catch up on his paper work. By his third day on only water he would be out doing hard physical chores like cutting the grass, splitting wood or weeding his vegetable garden. Day four would also be an energetic one, but if the fast extended beyond that, lowering blood sugar would begin to make him tired and he'd feel forced to begin laying down.

After a day of water fasting the average person's blood sugar level naturally drops; making a faster feel somewhat tired and "spacey," so a typical faster usually begins to spend much more time resting, further reducing the amount of energy being expended on moving the body around, serendipitously redirecting even more of the body's energy budget toward healing. By the end of five or six days on water, I estimate that from 40 to 50 percent of the body's available energy is being used for healing, repair and detoxification.

The amount of work that a fasting body's own healing energy can do and what it feels like to be there when it is happening is incredible. But you can't know it if you haven't felt it. So hardly anyone in our present culture knows.

As I mentioned in the first chapter, at Great Oaks School I apprenticed myself to the traveling masters of virtually every system of natural healing that existed during the '70s. I observed every one of them at work and tried most of them on my clients.

After all that I can say with experience that I am not aware of any other healing tool that can be so effective as the fast.

Essentials of a Successful, Safe Fast

1. Fast in a bright airy room, with exceptionally good ventilation, because fasters not only need a lot of fresh air; their bodies give off powerfully offensive odors.

Stacey L. Reid

2. Sun bathe if possible in warm climates for 10 to 20 minutes in the morning before the sun gets too strong.

3. Scrub/massage the skin with a dry brush, stroking toward the heart, followed by a warm water shower two to four times a day to assist the skin in eliminating toxins. If you are too weak to do this, have an assisted bed bath.

4. Have two enemas daily for the first week of a fast and then once daily until the fast is terminated.

5. Insure a harmonious environment with supportive people or else fast alone if you are experienced. Avoid well-meaning interference or anxious criticism at all cost. The faster becomes hypersensitive to others' emotions.

6. Rest profoundly except for a short walk of about 200 yards morning and night.

7. Drink water! At least three quarts every day. Do not allow yourself to become dehydrated!

8. Control yourself! Break a long fast on diluted non-sweet fruit juice such as grapefruit juice, sipped a teaspoon at a time, no more than eight ounces at a time no oftener than every 2 or 3 hours.

The second day you eat, add small quantities of fresh juicy fruit to the same amount of juice you took the day before no oftener than every 3 hours. By small quantities I mean half an apple or the equivalent. On the third day of eating, add small quantities of vegetable juice and juicy vegetables such as tomatoes and cucumbers. Control yourself! The second week after eating resumed add complex vegetable salads plus more complex fruit salads. Do not mix fruit and vegetables at meals. The third week add raw nuts and seeds no more than 1/2 ounce three times daily.

Home Remedies
Add 1/4 avocado daily. Fourth week increase to 3 ounces of raw soaked nuts and seeds daily and 1/2 avocado daily. Cooked grains may also be added, along with steamed vegetables and vegetable soups.

The Prime Rules of Fasting

Another truism of natural hygiene is that we dig our own graves with our teeth. It is sad but true that almost all eat too much quantity of too little quality. Dietary excesses are the main cause of death in North America. Fasting balances these excesses. If people were to eat a perfect diet and not overeat, fasting would rarely be necessary.

There are two essential rules of fasting. If these rules are ignored or broken, fasting itself can be life threatening. But if the rules are followed, fasting presents far less risk than any other important medical procedure with a far greater likelihood of a positive outcome. And let me stress here, there is no medical procedure without risk. Life itself is fraught with risk, it is a one-way ticket from birth to death, with no certainty as to when the end of the line will be reached. But in my opinion, when handling degenerative illness and infections, natural hygiene and fasting usually offer the best hope of healing with the least possible risk.

The first vital concern is the duration of the fast. Two eliminatory processes go on simultaneously while fasting. One is the dissolving and elimination of the excess, toxic or dysfunctional deposits in the body, and second process, the gradual exhaustion of the body's stored nutritional reserves. The fasting body first consumes those parts of the body that are unhealthy; eventually these are all gone. Simultaneously the body uses up stored fat and other reserve nutritional elements. A well-fed reasonably healthy body usually has enough stored nutrition too fast for quite a bit longer than it takes to "clean house."

While house cleaning is going on the body uses its reserves to rebuild organs and rejuvenate itself. Rebuilding starts out very slowly but the repairs increase at an ever-accelerating rate. The "overhaul" can last only until the body has no more reserves.

Because several weeks of fasting must pass by before the "overhaul" gets going full speed, it is wise to continue fasting as long as possible so as to benefit from as much rejuvenation as possible.

It is best not to end the fast before all toxic or dysfunctional deposits are eliminated, or before the infection is overcome, or before the cause for complaint has been healed. The fast must be ended when most of the body's essential-to-life stored nutritional reserves are exhausted. If the fast goes beyond this point, starvation begins. Then, fasting-induced organic damage can occur, and death can follow, usually several weeks later. Almost anyone not immediately close to death has enough stored nutrition to water fast for ten days to two weeks. Most reasonably healthy people have sufficient reserves to water fast for a month. Later I will explain how a faster can somewhat resupply their nutritional reserves while continuing to fast, and thus safely extend the fasting period.

The second essential concern has to do with adjusting the intensity of the fast. Some individuals are so toxic that the waste products released during a fast are too strong, too concentrated or too poisonous for the organs of elimination to handle safely, or to be handled within the willingness of the faster to tolerate the discomforts that toxic releases generate. The highly-toxic faster may even experience life-threatening symptoms such as violent asthma attacks. This kind of faster has almost certainly been dangerously ill before the fast began.

Home Remedies

Others, though not dangerously sick prior to fasting, may be nearly as toxic and though not in danger of death, they may not be willing to tolerate the degree of discomfort fasting can trigger. For this reason I recommend that if at all possible, before undertaking a fast the person eats mostly raw foods for two months and clean up all addictions. This will give the body a chance to detoxify significantly before the water fast is started, and will make water fasting much more comfortable. Seriously, dangerously ill people should only fast with experienced guidance, so the rapidity of their detoxification process may be adjusted to a lower level if necessary.

A fast of only one week can accomplish a significant amount of healing. Slight healing does occur on shorter fasts, but it is much more difficult to see or feel the results. Many people experience rapid relief from acute headache pain or digestive distress such as gas attacks, mild gallbladder pain, stomach aches, etc., after only one day's abstention from food. In one week of fasting a person can relieve more dangerous conditions such as arthritic pain, rheumatism, kidney pain, and many symptoms associated with allergic reactions. But even more fasting time is generally needed for the body to completely heal serious diseases. That's because eliminating life-threatening problems usually involve rebuilding organs that aren't functioning too well. Major rebuilding begins only after major detoxification has been accomplished, and this takes time.

Yes, even lost organ function can be partially or completely restored by fasting. Aging and age-related degeneration is progressive, diminishing organ functioning. Organs that make digestive enzymes secrete fewer enzymes. The degenerated immune system loses the ability to mobilize as effectively when the body is attacked. Liver and kidney efficiency declines. The adrenals tire becoming incapable of dumping massive amounts of stress-handling hormones or of repeating that effort time after time without considerable rest in between; the consequences of these inter-dependent deterioration's is a cascade of deterioration that contributes to even more rapid deterioration's. The name for this cascading process is aging. Its inevitable result--death.

Fasting can, to a degree, reverse aging. Because fasting improves organ functioning, it can slow down aging.

Fasters are often surprised that intensified healing can be uncomfortable. They have been programmed by our culture and by allopathic doctors to think that if they are doing the right thing for their bodies they should feel better immediately. I wish it weren't so, but most people have to pay the piper for their dietary indiscretions and other errors in living. There will be aches and minor pains and uncomfortable sensations. More about that later.

A rare faster does feel immediately better, and continues to feel ever better by the day, and even has incredible energy while eating nothing, but the majority of us folks just have to tough it out, keeping in mind that the way out is the way through. It is important to remind yourself at times that even with some discomfort and considering the inconvenience of fasting that you are getting off easy--one month of self-denial pays for those years of indulgence and buys a regenerated body.

Length of the Fast

How long should a person fast? In cases where there are serious complaints to remedy but where there are no life threatening disease conditions, a good rule of thumb is to fast on water for one complete day (24 hours) for each year that the person has lived. If you are 30 years old, it will take 30 consecutive days of fasting to restore complete health.

However, thirty fasting days, done a few days here and a few there won't equal a month of steady fasting; the body accomplishes enormously more in 7 or 14 days of consecutive fasting, than 7 or 14 days of fasting accumulated sporadically, such as one day a week. This is not to say that regular short fasts are not useful medicine. Periodic day-long fasts have been incorporated into many religious traditions, and for good reason; it gives the body one day a week to rest, to be free of digestive obligations, and to catch up on garbage disposal. I heartily recommend it. But it takes many years of unfailingly regular brief fasting to equal the benefits of one, intensive experience.

Fasting on water much longer than fifteen consecutive days may be dangerous for the very sick, (unless under experienced supervision) or too intense for those who are not motivated by severe illness to withstand the discomfort and boredom. However, it is possible to finish a healing process initiated by one long water fast by repeating the fast later. My husband's healing is a good example of this. His health began to noticeably decline about age 38 and he started fasting. He fasted on water 14 to 18 days at a time, once a year, for five consecutive years before most of his complaints and problems entirely vanished.

Common Fasting Complaints and Discomforts

The most frequently heard complaints of fasters are headaches, dry, cracked lips, dizziness, blurred vision with black spots that float, skin rashes, and weakness in the first few days plus what they think is intense hunger. The dizziness and weakness are really real, and are due to increased levels of toxins circulating in the blood and from unavoidably low blood sugar which is a natural consequence of the cessation of eating. The blood sugar does reestablish a new equilibrium in the second and third week of the fast and then, the dizziness may cease, but still, it is important to expect dizziness at the beginning.

It always takes more time for the blood to reach the head on a fast because everything has slowed down, including the rate of the heart beat, so blood pressure probably has dropped as well. If you stand up very quickly you may faint. I repetitively instruct all of my clients to stand up very slowly, moving from a lying to a sitting position, pausing there for ten or twenty seconds, and then rising slowly from a sitting to a standing position. They are told that at the first sign of dizziness they must immediately put their head between their knees so that the head is lower than the heart, or squat/sit down on the floor, I once had a faster who forgot to obey my frequent warnings.

About two weeks into a long fast, she got up rapidly from the toilet and felt dizzy. The obvious thing to do was to sit back down on the toilet or lie down on the bath rug on the floor, but no, she decided that because she was dizzy she should rush back to her bed in the adjoining room. She made it as far as the bathroom door and fainted, out cold, putting a deep grove into the drywall with her pretty nose on the way down. We then had to make an unscheduled visit to a nose specialist, who calmly put a tape-wrapped spoon inside her bent-over nose and pried it back to dead center. This was not much fun for either of us; it is well worthwhile preventing such complications.

Other common complaints during the fast include coldness, due to low blood sugar as well as a consequence of weight loss and slowed circulation due to lessened physical activity. People also dislike inactivity which seems excruciatingly boring, and some are upset by weight loss itself. Coldness is best handled with lots of clothes, bedding, hot water bottles or hot pads, and warm baths. Great Oaks School of Health was in Oregon, where the endlessly rainy winters are chilly and the concrete building never seemed to get really warm. I used to dream of moving my fasters to a tropical climate where I could also get the best, ripest fruits to wean them back on to food.

If the fast goes on for more than a week or ten days, many people complain of back discomfort, usually caused by over-worked kidneys. This passes. Hot baths or hot water bottles provide some relief.

Drinking more fluids may also help a bit. Nausea is fairly common too, due to toxic discharges from the gall bladder. Drinking lots of water or herbal tea dilutes toxic bile in the stomach and makes it more tolerable.

Very few fasters sleep well and for some reason they expect to, certainly fasters hope to, because they think that if they sleep all night they will better survive one more deadly dull day in a state of relative unconsciousness. They find out much to their displeasure that very little sleep is required on a fast because the body is at rest already. Many fasters sleep only two to four hours but doze frequently and require a great deal of rest. Being mentally prepared for this change of habit is the best handling. Generalized low-grade aches and pains in the area of the diseased organs or body parts are common and can often be alleviated with hot water bottles, warm but not hot bath water and massage. If this type of discomfort exists, it usually lessens with each passing day until it disappears altogether.

Many fasters complain that their vision is blurred, and that they are unable to concentrate. These are really major inconveniences because then fasters can't read or even pay close attention to video-taped movies, and if they can't divert themselves some fasters think they will go stir crazy. They are so addicted to a hectic schedule of doingness, and/or being entertained that they just can't stand just being with themselves, forced to confront and deal with the sensations of their own body, forced to face their own thoughts, to confront their own emotions, many of which are negative. People who are fasting release a lot of mental/emotional garbage at the same time as they let go of old physical garbage. Usually the psychological stuff contributed greatly to their illness and just like the physical garbage and degenerated organs, it all needs to be processed.

One of the most distressing experiences that happen occasionally is hair loss. Deprived of adequate nutrition, the follicles cannot keep growing hair, and the existing hair dies. However, the follicles themselves do not die and once the fast has ended and sufficient nutrition is forthcoming, hair will regrow as well or better than before.

There are also complaints that occur after the fast has been broken. Post-fast cravings, even after only two weeks of deprivation, are to be expected. These may take the form of desires for sweet, sour, salt, or a specific food dreamed of while fasting, like chocolate fudge Sundays or just plain toast. Food cravings must be controlled at all costs because if acted upon, each indulgence chips away the health gains of the previous weeks. A single indulgence can be remedied by a day of restricting the diet to juice or raw food.

After the repair, the person feels as good as they did when the fast ended. Repeated indulgences will require another extended bout of fasting to repair. It is far better to learn self-control.

Chapter 3- Is Colon Cleansing Good for You?

Colonics are one of the best types of medicine. They clean up deposits of old toxemia (though there are sure to be other deposits in the body's tissues colonics do not touch). Colon cleansing reduces the formation of new toxemia from putrefying fecal matter (but dietary reform is necessary to maximize this benefit). Most noticeable to the patient, a colonic immediately alleviates current symptoms by almost instantly reducing the current toxic load. A well-done enema or colonic is such a powerful technique that a single one will often make a severe headache vanish, make an onsetting cold go away, end a bout of sinusitis, end an asthmatic attack, reduce the pain of acute arthritic inflammation, reduce or stop an allergic reaction. Enemas are also thrifty: they are self-administered and can prevent most doctors' visits seeking relief for acute conditions.

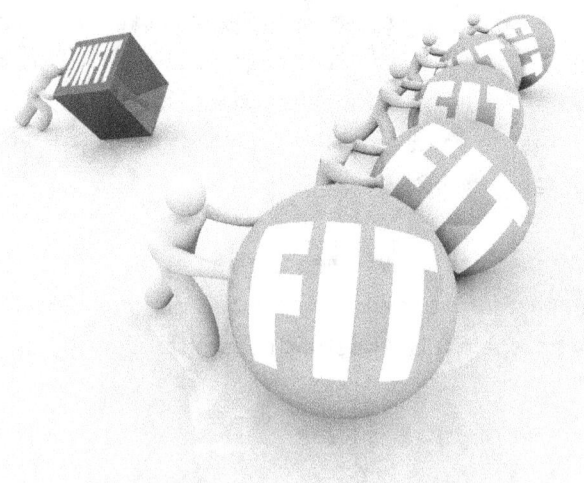

Diseases of the colon itself, including chronic constipation, colitis, diverticulitis, hemorrhoids, irritable bowel syndrome, and mucous colitis, are often cured solely by an intensive series of several dozen colonics given close together. Contrary to popular belief, many people think that if they have dysentery or other forms of loose stools that a colonic is the last thing they need.

Surprisingly, a series of colonics will eliminate many of these conditions as well. People with chronic diarrhea or loose stools are usually very badly constipated. This may seem a contradiction in terms but it will be explained shortly.

A century ago there was much less scientific data about the functioning of the human body. Then it was easy for a hygienically-oriented physician to come to believe that colonics were the single best medicine available. The doctor practicing nothing but colonics will have a very high rate of cure and a lot of very satisfied clients. Most importantly, this medicine will have done no harm.

The Repugnant Bowel

I don't know why, but people of our culture have a deep-seated reluctance to relate to the colon or its functions. People don't want to think about the colon or personally get involved with it by giving themselves enemas or colonics. They become deeply embarrassed at having someone else do it for them.

People are also shy about farts, and most persons have a hard time not smiling or reacting in some way when someone in their presence breaks wind, although the polite amongst us pretend that we didn't notice. Comedians usually succeed in getting a laugh out of an audience when they come up with a fart or make reference to some other bowel function. People don't react the same way to urinary functions or discharges, although these also may have an unpleasant odor and originate from the same "private" area.

Home Remedies

When I first mention to clients that they need a minimum of 12 colonics or many more enemas than 12 during a fasting or cleansing program they are inevitably shocked. To most it seems that no one in their right mind would recommend such a treatment, and that I must certainly be motivated by greed or some kind of a psychological quirk.

Then I routinely show them reproductions of X-rays of the large intestine showing obvious loss of normal structure and function resulting from a combination of constipation, the effects of gravity, poor abdominal muscle tone, emotional stress, and poor diet. In the average colon more than 50% of the hastrum (muscles that impel fecal matter through the organ) are dysfunctional due to loss of tone caused by impaction of fecal matter and/or constriction of the large intestine secondary to stress (holding muscular tension in the abdominal area) and straining during bowel movement.

A Typical Diseased Colon

The average person also has a prolapsed (sagging) transverse colon, and a distorted misplaced ascending and descending colon. I took a course in colon therapy before purchasing my first colonic machine. The chiropractor teaching the class required all of his patients scheduled for colonics to take a barium enema followed by an X-ray of their large intestine prior to having colonics and then make subsequent X-rays after each series of 12 colonics.

Most of his patients experienced so much immediate relief they voluntarily took at least four complete series, or 48 colonics, before their X-rays began to look normal in terms of structure. It also took about the same number, 48 colonics, for the patients to notice a significant improvement in the function of the colon. In reviewing over 10,000 X-rays taken at his clinic prior to starting colonics, the chiropractor had seen only two normal colon X-rays and these were from farm boys who grew up eating simple foods from the garden and doing lots of hard work.

The X-rays showed that it took a minimum of 12 colon treatments to bring about a minimal but observable change in the structure of the colon in the desired direction, and for the patient to begin to notice that bowel function was improving, plus the fact that they started to feel better.

Chapter 4- Diet and Nutrition

Appropriately new agey and spiritual, Macrobiotics teaches the way to perfect health is to eat like a Japanese whole foods vegetarian--the endless staple being brown rice, some cooked vegetables and seaweeds, meanwhile balancing the "yin" and "yang" of the foods. And Macrobiotics works great for a lot of people. But not all people. Because there's next to nothing raw in the Macrobiotic diet and some people are allergic to rice, or can get allergic to rice on that diet.

Linda Clark's Diet for a Small Planet also has hundreds of thousands of dedicated followers. This system balances the proportions of essential amino acids at every, single meal and is vegetarian. This diet also works and really helps some people, but not as well as Macrobiotics in my opinion because obsessed with protein, Clark's diet contains too many hard-to-digest soy products and makes poor food combinations from the point of digestive capacity.

Then there are the raw fooders. Most of them are raw, Organic fooders who go so far as to eat only unfired, unground cereals that have been soaked in warm water (at less than 115 degrees or you'll kill the enzymes) for many hours to soften the seeds up and start them sprouting. This diet works and really helps a lot of people.

Raw organic foodism is especially good for "holy joes," a sort of better-than-everyone-else person who enjoys great self-righteousness by owning this system. But raw fooding does not help all people nor solve all diseases because raw food irritates the digestive tracts of some people and in northern climates it is hard to maintain body heat on this diet because it is difficult to consume enough concentrated vegetable food in a raw state. And some raw fooders eat far too much fruit. I've seen them lose their teeth because of fruit's low mineral content, high sugar level and constant fruit acids in their mouths.

Then there are vegetarians of various varieties including vegans (vegetarians that will not eat dairy products and eggs), and then, there are their exact opposites, Atkins dieters focusing on protein and eating lots of meat. There's the Adelle Davis school, people eating whole grains, handfuls of vitamins, lots of dairy and brewers yeast and wheat germ, and even raw liver. Then there's the Organic school.

These folks will eat anything in any combination, just so long as it is organically produced, including organically raised beef, chicken, lamb, eggs, rabbit, wild meats, milk and dairy products, natural sea salt in large quantities and of course, organically grown fruits, vegetables grains and nuts. And what is "Organic?" The word means food raised in compliance with a set of rules contrived by a certification bureaucracy. When carefully analyzed, the somewhat illogical rules are not all that different in spirit than the rules of kashsruth or kosher. And the Organic certification bureaucrats aren't all that different than the rabbis who certify food as being kosher, either.

There are now millions of frightened Americans who, following the advice of mainstream Authority, have eliminated red meat from their diets and greatly reduced what they (mistakenly) understand as high-cholesterol foods.

All these diets work too--or some--and all demonstrate some of the truth.

The only area concerning health that contains more confusion and contradictory data than diet is vitamins. What a rats nest that is!

The Fundamental Principle

Home Remedies

If you are a true believer in any of the above food religions, I expect that you will find my views unsettling. But what I consider "good diet" results from my clinical work with thousands of cases. It is what has worked with those cases. My eclectic views incorporate bits and pieces of all the above. In my own case, I started out by following the Organic school, and I was once a raw food vegetarian who ate nothing but raw food for six years. I also ate Macrobiotic for about one year until I became violently allergic to rice.

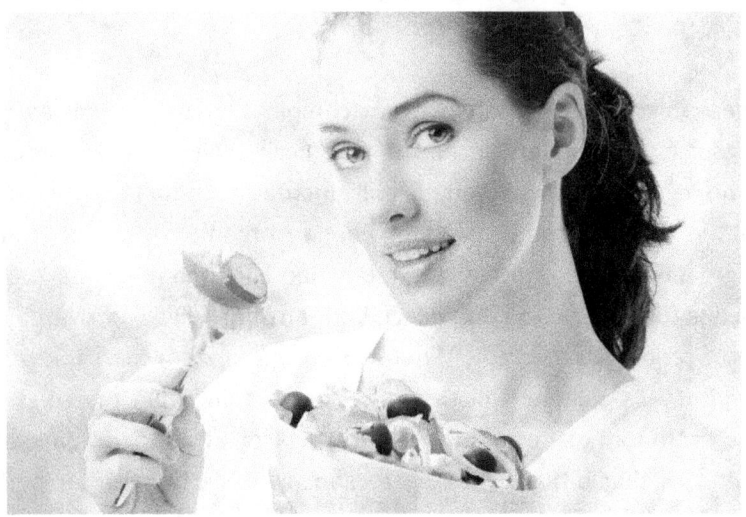

I have arrived at a point where I understand that each person's biochemistry is unique and each must work out their own diet to suit their life goals, life style, genetic predisposition and current state of health. There is no single, one, all-encompassing, correct diet. But, there is a single, basic, underlying Principle of Nutrition that is universally true. In its most simplified form, the basic equation of human health goes: Health = Nutrition / Calories. The equation falls far short of explaining the origin of each individuals diseases or how to cure diseases but Health = Nutrition/ Calories does show the general path toward healthful eating and proper medicine.

All animals have the exact same dietary problem: finding enough nutrition to build and maintain their bodies within the limits of their digestive capacity. Rarely in nature (except for predatory carnivores) is there any significant restriction on the number of calories or serious limitation of the amount of low-nutrition foods available to eat. There's rarely any shortage of natural junk food on Earth. Except for domesticated house pets, animals are sensible enough to prefer the most nutritional fare available and tend to shun empty calories unless they are starving.

But humans are perverse, not sensible. Deciding on the basis of artificially-created flavors, preferring insipid textures, we seem to prefer junk food and become slaves to our food addictions. For example, in tropical countries there is a widely grown root crop, called in various places: tapioca, manioc, or yuca. This interesting plant produces the greatest tonnage of edible, digestible, pleasant-tasting calories per acre compared to any other food crop I know. Manioc might seem the answer to human starvation because it will grow abundantly on tropical soils so infertile and/or so droughty that no other food crop will succeed there.

Manioc will do this because it needs virtually nothing from the soil to construct itself with. And consequently, manioc puts next to nothing nourishing into its edible parts. The bland-tasting root is virtually pure starch, a simple carbohydrate not much different than pure corn starch. Plants construct starches from carbon dioxide gas obtained the air and hydrogen obtained from water. There is no shortage ever of carbon from CO_2 in the air and rarely a shortage of hydrogen from water. When the highly digestible starch in manioc is chewed, digestive enzymes readily convert it into sugar.

Nutritionally there is virtually no difference between eating manioc and eating white sugar. Both are entirely empty calories.

Home Remedies

If you made a scale from ideal to worst regarding the ratio of nutrition to calories, white sugar, manioc and most fats are at the extreme undesirable end. Frankly I don't know which single food might lie at the extreme positive end of the scale. Close to perfect might be certain leafy green vegetables that can be eaten raw. When they are grown on extremely fertile soil, some greens develop 20 or more percent completely digestible balanced protein with ideal ratios of all the essential amino acids, lots of vitamins, tons of minerals, all sorts of enzymes and other nutritional elements--and very few calories. You could continually fill your stomach to bursting with raw leafy greens and still have a hard time sustaining your body weight if that was all you ate. Maybe Popeye the Sailorman was right about eating spinach.

For the moment, lets ignore individual genetic inabilities to digest specific foods and also ignore the effects stress and enervation can have on our ability to extract nutrition out of the food we are eating. Without those factors to consider, it is correct to say that, to the extent one's diet contains the maximum potential amount of nutrition relative to the number of calories you are eating, to that extent a person will be healthy. To the extent the diet is degraded from that ideal, to that extent, disease will develop.

Think about it!

CHAPTER 5- A LOOK AT FOOD SUPPLEMENTS

Sub-clinical, life-long, vitamin and mineral deficiencies contribute to the onset of disease; the malnourished body becomes increasingly enervated, beginning the process of disease. Vitamin supplements can increase the body's vital force, reversing to a degree the natural tendency towards degeneration. In fact, some medical gerontologists theorize that by using vitamins it might be possible to restore human life span to its genetically programmed 115 years without doing anything else about increasing nutrition from our degraded foods or paying much attention to dietary indiscretions. Knowing what I do about toxemia's effects I doubt vitamins can allow us to totally ignore what we eat, though supplements can certainly help.

More than degraded nutritional content of food prompts a thinking person to use food supplements. Our bodies and spirits are constantly assaulted and insulted by modern life in ways our genetics never intended us to deal with. Today the entire environment is mildly toxic. Air is polluted; water is polluted; our food supply contains traces of highly poisonous artificial molecules that our bodies have no natural ability to process and eliminate.

Our cities and work places are full of loud, shocking noises that trigger frequent adrenaline rushes and other stress adaptations. Our work places are full of psychological stresses that humans never had to deal with before.

Historically, humans who were not enslaved have been in control of determining their own hour to hour, day to day activities, living on their own largely self-sufficient farms. The idea of working for another, at regular hours, without personal liberty, ignoring or suppressing one's own agenda and inclinations over an entire lifetime is quite new and not at all healthy. It takes continual subconscious applications of mental and psychic energies to protect ourselves against the stresses of modern life, energies that we don't know we're expending. This is also highly enervating. Thus to remain healthy we may need nutrition at levels far higher than might be possible through eating food; even ideal food might not contain enough vitamins to sustain us against the strains and stresses of this century.

Compared to prescriptions, even the most exotic life extension supplements are much less expensive. I am saddened when my clients tell me they can't afford supplements. When their MD prescribes a medicine that costs many times more they never have trouble finding the money.

I am also saddened that people are so willing to take supplements, because I can usually do a lot more to genuinely help their bodies heal with dietary modification and detoxification. Of all the tools at my disposal that help people heal, last in the race come supplements.

One of the best aspects of using vitamins as though they were healing agents is that food supplements almost never have harmful side effects, even when they are taken in what might seem enormous overdoses. If someone with a health condition reads or hears about some vitamin being curative, goes out and buys some and takes it, they will at very least have followed the basic principle of good medicine: first of all do no harm.

At worst, if the supplements did nothing for them at all, they are practicing the same kind of benevolent medicine that Dr. Jennings did almost two centuries ago. Not only that, but having done something to treat their symptoms, they have become patients facilitating their own patience, giving their body a chance to correct its problem. They well may get better, but not because of the action of the particular vitamin they took. Or, luckily, the vitamin or vitamins they take may have been just what was needed, raising their body's vital force and accelerating the body's ability to solve its problem.

One reason vitamin therapies frequently do not work as well as they might is that, having been intimidated by AMA propaganda that has created largely false fears in the public mind about harmful effects of vitamin overdoses, the person may not take enough of the right vitamin. The minimum daily requirements of vitamins and minerals as outlined in nutrition texts are only sufficient to prevent the most obvious forms of deficiency diseases. If a person takes supplements at or near the minimum daily requirement (the dose recommended by the FDA as being 'generally recognized as safe') they should not expect to see any therapeutic effect unless they have scurvy, beri beri, rickets, goiter, or pellagra.

In these days of vitamin-fortified bread and iodized salt, and even vitamin C fortified soft drinks, you almost never see the kind of life-threatening deficiency states people first learned to recognize, such as scurvy. Sailors on long sea voyages used to develop a debilitating form of vitamin C deficiency that could kill. Scurvy could be quickly cured by as little as one lime a day.

For this reason the British Government legislated the carrying of limes on long voyages and today that is why British sailors are still called limeys. A lime has less than 30 milligrams of vitamin C. But to make a cold clear up faster with vitamin C a mere 30 mg does absolutely nothing! To begin to dent an infection with vitamin C takes 10,000 milligrams a day, and to make a life threatening infection like pneumonia go away faster might require 25,000 to 150,000 milligrams of vitamin C daily, administered intravenously.

Home Remedies

In terms of supplying that much C with limes, that's 300 to 750 of them daily--clearly impossible.

Similarly, pellagra can be cured with a few milligrams of vitamin B3, but schizophrenia can sometimes be cured with 3,000 milligrams, roughly a thousand times as much as the MDR.

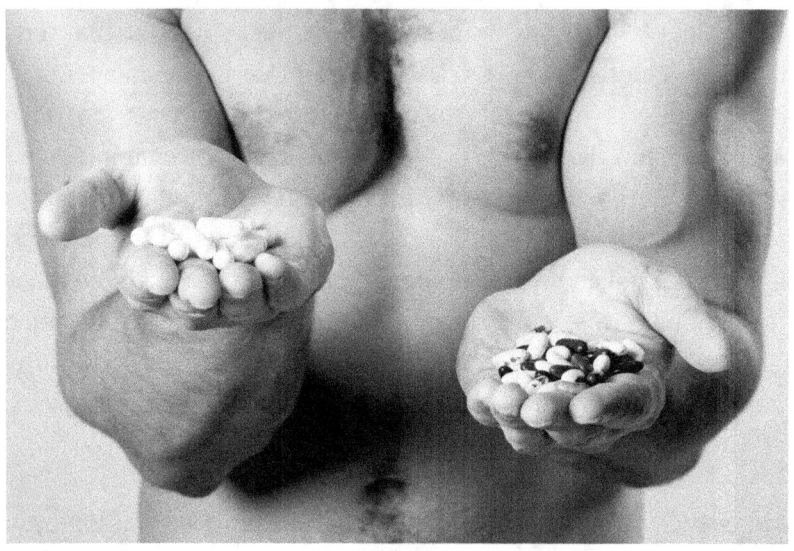

There are many common diseases that the medical profession does not see as being caused by vitamin deficiencies. Senility and many mental disorders fall in this category. Many old people live on extremely deficient diets comprised largely of devitalized starches, sugars, and fats, partly because many do not have good enough teeth to chew vegetables and other high roughage foods, and they do not have the energy it takes to prepare more nourishing foods. Virtually all old people have deficiency diseases. As vital force inevitably declines with age, the quantity and quality of digestive enzymes decreases, then the ability to breakdown and extract soluble nutrients from food is diminished, frequently leading to serious deficiencies. These deficiencies are inevitably misdiagnosed as disease and as aging.

Suppose a body needs 30 milligrams a day of niacin to not develop pellagra, but to be fully healthy, needs 500 milligrams daily. If that body receives 50 milligrams per day from a vitamin pill, to the medical doctor it could not possibly be deficient in this vitamin.

There is a big difference between preventing a gross vitamin deficiency disease, and using vitamins to create optimum functioning. Any sick person or anyone with a health complaint needs to improve their overall functioning in any way that won't be harmful over the long term. Vitamin therapy can be an amazingly effective adjunct to dietary reform and detoxification.

Some of the earlier natural hygienists were opposed to using

vitamins. However, these doctors lived in an era when the food supply was better, when mass human degeneration had not proceeded as far as it has today. From their perspective, it was possible to obtain all the nutrition one needed from food. In our time this is unlikely unless a person knowingly and intelligently produces virtually all their own food on a highly fertile soil body whose fertility is maintained and adjusted with a conscious intent to maximize the nutritive content of the food. Unfortunately, ignorance of the degraded nature of industrial food seems to extend to otherwise admirable natural healing methods such as Macrobiotics and homeopathy because these disciplines also downplay any need for food supplementation.

Vitamins for Young Persons and Children

Young healthy people from weaning through their thirties should also take nutritional supplements even though young people usually feel so good that they find it impossible to conceive that anything could harm them or that they ever could become seriously sick or actually die. I know this is true because I remember my own youth and besides, why else would young people so glibly ride motorcycles or, after only a few months of brainwashing, charge up a hill into the barrel of a machine gun. Or have unsafe sex in this age of multiple venereal diseases.

Until they get a little sense, vitamin supplements help to counteract their inevitable and unpreventable use of recreational foods. Vitamins are the cheapest long life and health insurance plan now available. Parents are generally very surprised at the thought that even their children need nutritional supplements; very few healthy children receive them. A few are given extra vitamin C when acutely ill, when they have colds or communicable diseases such as chicken pox.

Young people require a low dose supplement compared to those of us middle-aged or older, but it should be a broad formula with the full range of vitamins and minerals.

Healthy very small children who will swallow pills can take the same products at half the recommended dose. If they won't swallow pills the pills can be blended into a fruit smoothie or finely crushed and then stirred into apple sauce.

Vitamins for an Older Healthy Person

Someone who is beyond 35 to 40 years of age should still feel good almost all of the time. That is how life should be. But enjoying well-being does not mean that no dietary supplementation is called for. The onset of middle age is the appropriate time to begin working on continuing to feel well for as long as possible. Just like a car, if you take very good care of it from the beginning, it is likely to run smoothly for many years into the future.

If on the other hand you drive it hard and fast with a lot of deferred maintenance you will probably have to trade it in on a new one after a very few years. Most people in their 70s and older who are struggling with many uncomfortable symptoms and low energy lament, 'if I'd only known I was going to live so long I would have taken better care of myself.' But at that point it is too late for the old donkey; time for a trade in.

Vitamin supplements can actually slow or even to a degree, reverse, the aging process. However, to accomplish that task, they have to be taken in amounts far greater than so-called minimum daily requirements, using vitamins as though they were drugs, a therapeutic approach to changing body chemistry profiles and making them resemble a younger body. For example, research gerontologists like Walford reason that if pantothenic acid (vitamin B5), in fairly substantial (but quite safe) doses can extend the life and improve the function of old rats, there is every indication that it will do a similar job on humans. Medical researchers and research gerontologists have noticed that many other vitamin and vitamin-like substances have similar effects on laboratory animals.

The Future of Life Extension

I beg the readers indulgence for a bit of futurology about what things may look like if the life extension movement continues to develop.

Right now, a full vitamin and vitamin-like substance life extension program costs between $50 and $100 dollars per month. However, pharmaceutical researchers occasionally notice that drugs meant to treat and cure diseases, when tested on lab animals for safety, make these animals live quite a bit longer and function better. Though the FDA doesn't allow any word of this to be printed in official prescribing data, the word does get around to other researchers, to gerontologists and eventually to that part of the public that is eagerly looking for longer life. Today there are numerous people who routinely take prescription medicines meant to cure a disease they do not have and plan to take those medicines for the rest of their long, long life.

Vitamin Program for the Sick

No matter which way you look at it or how well insured you may be against it, being sick is expensive (not to mention what it does to one's quality of life), and by far the best thing to do is to prevent it from happening in the first place. However, most people do not do anything about their health until forced to by some painful condition. If you are already sick there are a number of supplements you can take which have the potential to shorten the duration and severity of the illness, and hopefully prevent a recurrence.

The sicker you are the more supplements you will require; as health is regained, the dosage and variety of substances can be reduced. In chronic illness, megadoses of many nutrients are usually beneficial. Any sick adult should begin a life extension vitamin program unless they are highly allergic to so many things already that they cannot tolerate many kinds of vitamins as well. In addition to the life extension program, vitamin C should be taken by the chronically ill at a dose from 10 to 25 grams daily, depending on the severity of the condition.

Many people want to know whether or not they should take their regular food supplements during a fast. On a water fast most supplements in a hard tablet form will not be broken down at all, and often can be seen floating by in the colonic viewing tube looking exactly like it did when you swallowed it. This waste can be avoided by crushing or chewing (yuck) the tablets, before swallowing. Encapsulated vitamins usually are absorbed, but if you want to make sure, open the capsule and dump it in the back of your mouth before swallowing with water. Powdered vitamins are well absorbed.

On a water fast the body is much more sensitive to any substance introduced, so as a general rule it is not a good idea to take more than one half your regular dose of food supplements. Most fasters do fine without any supplements. Many people get an upset stomach from supplements on an empty stomach, and these people should not take any during a water fast unless they develop symptoms of mineral deficiencies (usually a pre-existing condition) such as leg cramps and tremors, these symptoms necessitate powdered or well-chewed-up mineral supplement. Minerals don't taste too bad to chew, just chalky.

The same suggestions regarding dosage of supplements for a water fast are also true for a juice fast or vegetable broth fast. On a raw food cleansing diet the full dose of supplements should be taken with meals.

There exists an enormous body of data about vitamins; books and magazine articles are always touting some new product or explaining the uses of an old one. If you want to know more about using ordinary vitamins you'll find leads in the bibliography to guide your reading. However, there is one "old" vitamin and a few newer and relatively unknown life extending substances that are so useful and important to handling illness that I would like to tell you more about them.

Vitamin C is not a newly discovered vitamin, but was one of the first ever identified. If you are one of those people that just hate taking vitamins, and you were for some reason willing to take only one, vitamin C would be your best choice. Vitamin C would be the clear winner because it helps enormously with any infection and in invaluable in tissue healing and rebuilding collagen. If I was going on a long trip and didn't want to pack a lot of weight, my first choice would be to insure three to six grams of vitamin C for daily use when I was healthy (I'd take the optimum dose--ten grams a day--if weight were no limitation). I'd also carry enough extra C to really beef up my intake when dealing with an unexpected acute illness or accident.

When traveling to faraway places, exposed to a whole new batch of organisms, frequently having difficulty finding healthy foods, going through time zones, losing nights of sleep, it is easy to become enervated enough to catch a local cold or flu. If I have brought lots of extra vitamin C with me I know that my immune system will be able to conquer just about anything--as long as I also stop eating and can take an enema. I also like to have vitamin C as a part of my first aid kit because if I experience a laceration, a sprain, broken bone, or a burn, I can increase my internal intake as well as apply it liberally directly on the damaged skin surface. Vitamin C can be put directly in the eye in a dilute solution with distilled water for infections and injuries, in the ear for ear infections, and in the nose for sinus infections. If you are using the acid form of C (ascorbic acid) and it smarts too much, make a more dilute solution, or switch to the alkaline form of C (calcium ascorbate) which can be used as a much more concentrated solution without a stinging sensation. Applied directly on the skin C in solution makes a very effective substitute for sun screen. It doesn't filter out ultraviolet, it beefs up the skin to better deal with the insult.

I believe vitamin C can deal with a raging infection such as pneumonia as well or better than antibiotics. But to do that, C is going to have to be administered at the maximum dose the body can process. This is easily discoverable by a 'bowel tolerance test' which basically means you keep taking two or three grams of C each hour, (preferably in the powdered, most rapidly assimilable form) until you get a runny stool (the trots). The loose stool happens when there is so much C entering the small intestine that it is not all absorbed, but is instead, passed through to the large

Stacey L. Reid

intestine. At that point cut back just enough that the stool is only a little loose, not runny. At this dose, your blood stream will be as saturated by vitamin C as you can achieve by oral ingestion.

It can make an important difference which type of vitamin C is taken because many people are unable to tolerate the acid form of C beyond 8 or 10 grams a day, but they can achieve a therapeutic dose without discomfort with the alkaline (buffered) vitamin C products such as calcium ascorbate, sodium ascorbate, or magnesium-potassium ascorbates.

Vitamin C also speeds up the healing of internal tissues and damaged connective tissue. Damaged internal tissues might include stomach ulcers (use the alkaline form of vitamin C only), bladder and kidney infections (acid form usually best), arthritic disorders with damage to joints and connective tissue (alkaline form usually best). Sports injuries heal up a lot faster with a therapeutic dose of vitamin C. As medicine, vitamin C should be taken at the rate of one or two grams every two hours (depending on the severity of the condition), spaced out to avoid unnecessary losses in the urine which happens if it were taken ten grams at a time. If you regularly use the acid form of vitamin C powder, which is the cheapest, be sure to use a straw and dissolve it in water or juice so that the acid does not dissolve the enamel on your teeth over time.

Co-enzyme Q-10

This substance is normally manufactured in the human body and is also found in minuscule amounts in almost every cell on Earth. For that reason it is also called "ubiquinone." But this vitamin has been only recently discovered, so as I write this book Co-enzyme Q-10 is not widely known.

Home Remedies

Q-10 is essential to the functioning of the mitochondria, that part of the cell that produces energy. With less Q-10 in heart cells, for example, the heart has less energy and pumps less. The same is true of the immune system cells, the liver cells, every cell. As we age the body is able to make less and less Q-10, contributing to the loss of energy frequently experienced with age, as well as the diminished effectiveness of the immune system, and a shortened life span.

Q-10 was first used for its ability to revitalize heart cells. It was a prescription medicine in Japan. But unlike other drugs used to stimulate the heart, at any reasonable dose Q-10 has no harmful side effects. It also tends to give people the extra pick up they are trying to get out of a cup of coffee. But Q-10 does so by improving the function of every cell in the body, not by whipping exhausted adrenals like caffeine does. Q-10 is becoming very popular with athletes who measure their overall cellular output against known standards.

Besides acting as a general tonic, when fed to lab animals, Co-Enzyme Q-10 makes them live 33 to 45 percent longer!

DMAE is another extremely valuable vitamin-like substance that is not widely known. It is a basic building material that the body uses to make acetylcholine, the most generalized neurotransmitter in the body. Small quantities of DMAE are found in fish, but the body usually makes it in a multi-stage synthesis that starts with the amino acid choline, arrives at DMAE at about step number three and ends up finally with acetylcholine.

The body's nerves are wrapped in fatty tissue that should be saturated with acetylcholine. Every time a nerve impulse is transmitted from one nerve cell to the next, a molecule of acetylcholine is consumed. Thus acetylcholine has to be constantly replaced. As the body ages, levels of acetylcholine surrounding the nerves drop and in consequence, the nerves begin to deteriorate. DMAE is rapidly and easily converted into acetylcholine and helps maintain acetylcholine levels in older people at a youthful level.

When laboratory rats are fed DMAE they solve mazes more rapidly, remember better, live about 40 percent longer than rats not fed DMAE and most interestingly, when autopsied, their nervous systems resemble those of a young rat, without any evidence of the usual deterioration of aging. Human nervous systems also deteriorate with age, especially those of people suffering from senility. It is highly probable that DMAE will do the same thing to us. DMAE also smoothes out mood swings in humans and seems to help my husband, Steve, when he has a big writing project. He can keep working without getting 'writers block', fogged out, or rollercoastering.

DMAE is a little hard to find. Prolongevity and VRP sell it in powder form. Since the FDA doesn't know any MDR and since the product is not capped up, the bottle of powder sagely states that one-quarter teaspoonful contains 333 milligrams. Get the hint? DMAE tastes a little like sour salt and one-quarter teaspoonful dissolves readily in water every morning before breakfast, or anytime for that matter. DMAE is also very inexpensive considering what it does. A year's supply costs about $20.

Lecithin is a highly tonic and inexpensive food supplement that is underutilized by many people even though it is easily obtainable in healthfood stores. It is an emulsifier, breaking fats down into small separate particles, keeping blood cholesterol emulsified to prevent arterial deposits. Taken persistently, lecithin partially and slowly eliminates existing cholesterol deposits from the circulatory system.

In our cholesterol-frightened society lecithin should be a far more popular supplement than it currently is. It is easy to take either as a food in the granular form or when encapsulated. Lecithin granules have very little flavor and can be added to a home-made vinegar and oil salad dressing, where they emulsify the oil and make it blend with the vinegar, thickening the mixture and causing it to stick to the salad better. Lecithin can also be put in a fruits smoothie. A scant tablespoon a day is sufficient. Try to buy the kind of lecithin that has the highest phosphatidyl choline content because this substance is the second benefit of taking lecithin.

Phosphatidyl choline is another precursor used by the body to build acetylcholine and helps maintain the nervous system.

Algae. Spirulina or sun dried chlorella are also great food supplements. Both make many people feel energized, pepped-up. It is possible to fast on either product and still maintain sufficient energy levels to take of minimal work responsibilities. Algae reduces appetite and as a dietary supplement can assist in weight loss. It contains large amounts of protein due to its high chlorophyll content, as well as a large amount of beta carotene. It also assists in detoxification of the lymphatic system. It can be purchased as tablets or powder. Take a heaping teaspoon daily, or at least six tablets.

ABOUT THE AUTHOR

Stacey L. Reid has long been interested in home remedies and the validity of the studies that have been done on them. She has done extensive research on herbal remedies, aromatherapy and other alternate forms of treatment. Her latest book is extremely complex and explores a lot of the alternate theories surrounding health and wellness.

She is currently getting certified as a nutritionist so that she will be better able to help her own family and others to eat properly.